You Can Do the Splits!

Scientific Stretching
for
Fast Results!

Everything You Need to Know to
Achieve Maximum Flexibility as
Quickly, Safely and Efficiently as Possible!

Jon Deva

DEDICATION

This book is dedicated to you, dear reader. You have sought out this valuable information and now all you have to do is learn it and apply it.
Kudos to you! I wish you success in this and all your endeavors.

Medical Disclaimer

Always consult your physician before beginning any exercise program. This general information is not intended to diagnose any medical condition or to replace your healthcare professional.

Never disregard professional medical advice or delay in seeking it because of something you have read in this or any other publication. Any content or information provided herein is for informational and educational purposes only and any use thereof is solely at your own risk. The author and publisher bears no responsibility thereof.

The information contained herein is not intended to be a substitute for professional medical advice, diagnosis or treatment in any manner. Always seek the advice of your physician or other qualified health provider with any questions you may have regarding any medical condition. All information contained in this publication is for informational and educational purposes only.

CONTENTS

1

How this information was Collected/Researched/Discovered

When I was a teenager, I started training in Kung Fu classes and doing yoga every day. In Kung Fu, everybody does warm-ups and stretches at the beginning of class. In yoga, the entire class is devoted to stretching and assuming stretched postures. Yet in both of those classes, I noticed that some people were naturally flexible and that others never seemed to make any gains in flexibility whatsoever, despite day after day, month after month of practicing. If you have ever participated in a yoga or martial arts class for any period of time, you have probably noticed the same thing in yourself and others.

I did OK with my stretching. I was able to do a decent forward bend and I could kick high pretty easily, with my legs opening to about 160 degrees. But the full splits and those perfectly vertical kicks that the Chinese Kung Fu guys did in the movies seemed impossible to reach. Were they just naturally flexible? What were their training methods? I decided to look into it.

In China, martial arts training goes back thousands of years and Chinese people seem to have lots and lots of time on their hands. At a wushu school in china, you will typically find the students doing warm-up stretches for a full TWO HOURS before they begin their actual kicking and punching routines that they spend the next six hours on.

So that was the way they did it. Just put in a full two hours of stretching every day and in a few weeks or months depending on your age you will reach your maximum potential. That was the Chinese way.

Well, although I was dedicated to training, I didn't want to spend two hours of everyday stretching. I had school to go to, work to do, and I wanted to have some time left to actually train in martial arts!

So I continued to search.

I discovered that many scientific studies on flexibility had been done in Russia by government sponsored scientists in the interest of improving their Olympic athletes. These studies were a gold mine of information. The Russian scientists tested everything, different kinds of stretching, different frequencies of stretching, different intensities of stretching, length of time in position, number of repetitions, etc. They tested every possible variable to find out what the best methods of improving flexibility actually were. There was a tremendous amount of information there, but I had to sort through all the studies and analyze the data to determine what variables had produced the best results.

What I discovered was that there were two kinds of stretching that had produced the best results in the shortest amount of time.

I learned the techniques, applied both of the methods to my practice and in a short period of time, I was able to do the full splits, in every direction, quite easily. So now here I am, 30 years later, still strong and flexible, and I have decided to share my secrets of strength and flexibility with you!

I am very happy and excited to share this method with you, and I'm sure you will be very excited and pleased with the results as you learn how easily and quickly you can achieve the flexibility you have always dreamed of.

I'll See you in the next Chapter.

2

Understanding Methods of Stretching

Welcome to the section on Understanding Methods of Stretching.

The first thing to understand is that while at first it may seem to be a simple thing, there are many, many methods of stretching. Depending on how you decide to divide them up, you can say there are six, eight, or even twelve or more methods of stretching.

We are not going to cover them all, and the pros and cons of each, in this book. I may produce an in-depth course in the future for personal trainers and coaches, but this book is the quick and dirty, how to get in the splits as fast as possible course, so we only need to talk about three kinds of stretching.

The three kinds of stretching we will learn about now are:

Static, **Dynamic**, and **PNF** stretching, which is also known as **Contract/Relax/Extend** stretching.

What follows is an introduction and overview of each of these three types.

1: Static Stretching

2: Dynamic Stretching

3: PNF- Contract/Relax/Extend Stretching

Let's begin:

Static Stretching

We're going to start by talking about static stretching because it is the most well-known and common form of stretching. We will learn exactly what it is, how most people do it, what's wrong with how most people do it, common mistakes, what it is actually good for, and how and when to do it correctly. Static stretching is actually not a focus of this course, but it is necessary to understand it completely, how to do it right, and how it is different from the other types of stretching that we will be utilizing to get into the splits fast.

What it is:

Common Static Stretching can more specifically be called **Static Passive Relaxed** Stretching. This is because the way that static stretching is usually done is by moving a muscle to the far limit of its range of motion, then relaxing the muscle and just holding the position for a period of time.

For example, to stretch the back of the leg, you might lift your leg onto a bar or horizontal surface, stretching the leg out straight and then just holding the position, with the muscles on the back of the leg stretched, but relaxed as possible. Since the weight of the leg is supported, both the muscles on the front and back of the leg are relaxed. That's what makes it

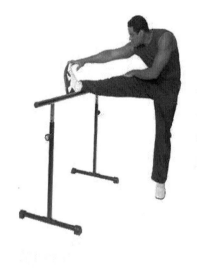

"**Passive Relaxed**". And of course, you are not moving, so that's what makes it "**Static**".

Or, you might be seated on the ground with your legs spread as far apart as possible. You then bend forward between the legs and over the legs and hold the position. In this stretch you are attempting to stretch the muscles on the back of the leg and the inside of the leg. Since you are supported by the floor, all of these muscles remain relaxed, and you just hold the position. You are not moving, so the pose is **Static**, and all the muscles being stretched are **Passive** and **Relaxed**.

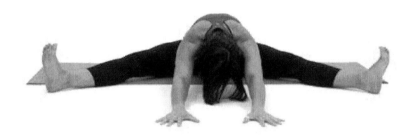

So this is the kind of stretching most people are familiar with and most people do when they go to the gym to begin some type of workout. So why don't people get more flexible using this method? What's wrong with it? Usually lots of things…

First of all, static stretching should not be done at the beginning of workouts! While it is common in many schools, athletic traditions and military practices to do static stretching before running or workouts, it serves no purpose to stretch cold muscles and is in fact detrimental. It increases the chance of injury by temporarily decreasing the sensitivity of the nerves in the muscles being stretched. This is quite obvious to anyone who does a deep static stretch of the legs, then gets up and tries to walk. The legs will feel a little wobbly.

5

Static stretching should be performed at the end of workouts, on warmed up muscles.

The next common problem with static stretching is that people don't usually hold the position long enough to achieve the desired effect. They might hold the position for ten or twenty seconds, then switch to the other leg, and then repeat. That is simply not long enough. To receive any benefit from static stretching, you must hold the position for an absolute minimum of 30 seconds. One minute is even better.

The reason is because it takes about 45 seconds to a full minute of stretch to override the Stretch Reflex and the Golgi Tendon Reflex systems of your body. The Stretch Reflex and the Golgi Tendon Reflex are two aspects of your nervous system that are designed to protect you from injury. Your body possesses great wisdom and it is always trying to protect you. We don't need to study these two reflexes in detail here. Just know that in order for static stretching to have any benefit whatsoever in reprogramming the nervous system, you have to hold the stretch for 45 to 60 seconds. Look at a watch or clock while you are static stretching, 45 seconds to one minute is longer than most people think!

Static stretches should be held for 45 seconds to one minute at a time.

The next common problem with static stretching is that people do not relax enough in the position. It is important to consciously relax the muscle being stretched. While watching the clock to make sure you hold the position long enough, you breathe deeply and slowly and concentrate your mind on relaxing the muscle that is being stretched.

Breathe deeply and slowly and consciously relax the muscle being stretched.

Another common problem with static stretching is that many people push the limit too hard. When moving your limbs toward the end of your current range of motion, you start to feel the stretch, then it feels a bit difficult, then it can hurt. People think that they need to push to the maximum to extend their stretch, and they push too hard. The result is that the muscles become sore, and instead of lengthening, they become tighter. If your muscles are extremely sore the day after static stretching, you have pushed too far. The "No Pain, No Gain" theory of exercise does not apply to stretching! There should never be any pain involved in any stretching method. Ever!

This hurts, but I've got to push my limits! WRONG!

This is getting difficult...   This is the correct zone!

This feels like a stretch.   Feels good, but doesn't acomplish anything.

The proper way is to extend to that middle section, after you start to feel the stretch, and before it hurts. That is where you hold the static position for 45 to 60 seconds.

Never cause pain! It doesn't help and only hinders your efforts. Push only to the difficult level.

Static Stretching: Summary

So we've learned a bit about static stretching and some of the things people do wrong, and why they don't get good results. Even if you do everything right, you may not get the best results from **Static Passive Relaxed** stretching. The truth is, this kind of stretching is really not very good at increasing your flexibility.

So what is it good for? How, when, and why should **Static Passive Relaxed** stretching be done? Let's talk about that now:

Static Stretching: The Right Way

- The proper time to perform static stretching is at the end of a workout, on warmed-up muscles.

- The proper way to perform static stretching is to assume the stretched position, just to where it gets difficult, not causing pain, relax and breathe and hold the position for 45 to 60 seconds.

- The purpose of static stretching is to re-align the muscle fibers that may have become knotted or twisted as they become fatigued during intense physical activity and to keep the muscle from shortening, losing the flexibility you already have.

- Static stretching is time consuming and a poor choice for increasing your range of motion, however should be done for the reason stated above.

- Static stretching is optional, and not emphasized in this course for the reasons stated earlier.

- We have learned about static stretching here so we can understand the difference between static stretching and the two methods that follow in the next chapters.

3

Dynamic Stretching

Dynamic Stretching is moving a limb back and forth between the full range of motion currently possible for the limb. Although there is movement, the limb being stretched is kept as relaxed as possible.

Examples of **Dynamic Stretching** you may be familiar with are: arm circles, arm swings for the chest, and leg swinging for the hips and hamstrings.

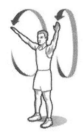 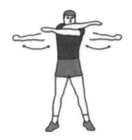 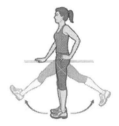

Most people think of these kinds of movements only as warm-ups, but they are both warming up and stretching the muscle groups in question.

In **Dynamic Stretching**, the speed of movement changes as the muscles get warmed up. One begins by gently and slowly moving the limb through the range of motion, then speeding up as the muscles warm up and stay relaxed. The range of motion will gradually increase as the muscles get warmed up and accustomed to the exercise. Although the speed increases, the limb stays as relaxed as possible.

Dynamic Stretching has proven itself to be much more efficient than static stretching at increasing flexibility, both dynamic and static.

In this quick course on achieving the splits as fast as possible, we will be concentrating on leg swinging stretches as our primary **Dynamic** stretch.

We will be swinging the legs in three directions. In two of those directions, we will be stopping the leg at the top of the range of motion with our hands or a padded object. This encourages the muscles to relax.

Exact details follow in later sections.

Dynamic vs. Ballistic

You may have heard of ballistic stretching (which everyone says not to do) and wondering what the difference is between Dynamic Stretching and Ballistic Stretching.

Dynamic Stretching differs from **Ballistic Stretching** in the following ways:

Ballistic Stretching is performed at high speed, kicking the leg up as fast as possible.	**Dynamic** Stretching starts slow, then medium, then faster speeds.
Ballistic Stretching allows the limb to bang against the end of the range of motion at high speed, forcefully stretching the muscle which is under tension.	In my method of **Dynamic** Stretching, the limb is stopped at the high end of the range of motion by your hands or a padded object, allowing the stretched muscle to relax, as it is not responsible for stopping the movement of the limb.

4

PNF - Contract/Relax/Extend Stretching

What the heck is **PNF Stretching**? **PNF stretching**, or proprioceptive neuromuscular facilitation stretching, is a set of stretching techniques commonly used in clinical and athletic environments to enhance both active and passive range of motion with the ultimate goal being to optimize range of motion and motor performance.

This type of stretching, when done properly, **has been proven to make the fastest gains in range of motion in a short period of time when done correctly.** Aside from being safe and time efficient, the dramatic gains in range of motion seen in a short period of time is motivating and keeps you going with the program.

There are many variations of **PNF Stretching**. In this course of achieving the splits as quickly and efficiently as possible, we use the **Contract/Relax/Extend** technique.

To begin the method of **PNF Stretching,** you move a limb to the end of its current range of motion and support it, just like static stretching the leg on a horizontal bar. In static stretching, we just leave the leg on the bar and relax the muscles of the leg and hold the position for a period of time.

In **PNF Stretching**, we start off this way and then we add specific cycles of contraction and relaxation of the muscles being stretched.

So, for example, you would place the leg on the bar, toes pointing up to stretch the hamstrings on the back of the leg. With the leg in this position, you then consciously contract the muscles on the back of the leg, pushing down on the bar, for 8-10 seconds, then you relax the muscles completely for 20-30 seconds. At this point, you usually find that your range of motion has increased a little, so you extend the stretch a little further and begin the cycle again. This is repeated a total of 3 times.

1: Stretch - Contract 8-10 seconds – Relax 20-30 seconds – Extend Range of Motion a little bit

2: Stretch - Contract 8-10 seconds – Relax 20-30 seconds – Extend Range of Motion a little bit

3: Stretch - Contract 8-10 seconds – Relax 20-30 seconds – Extend Range of Motion a little bit

That is how the **Contract/Relax/Extend Stretching** is done.

Notes:

➢ During the 8-10 second contraction, the muscle should be contracted only to 50% to 75% of full tension. Do not contract maximally.

➢ There is (usually) no benefit in repeating the cycle more than three times.

➢ Sometimes, your muscles will be tight and refuse to extend. Do not force increased range of motion.

➢ **PNF Stretching** is only to be done 3 times per week.

➢ **PNF Stretching** will produce some amount of muscle soreness on the following day. You should know that you stretched the night before, but you should not be in pain and unable to walk. If so, you over did it!

Exact details on the **PNF Stretching** techniques used in this course will follow in later chapters.

5

Summary - 3 Types of Stretching Used in this Course

So, we have learned about three types of stretching now, static stretching, dynamic stretching, and PNF stretching.

We have learned that static stretching is not really part of this course, but we should do static stretching at the end of our workouts to maintain flexibility and re-align the muscle fibers that may have become knotted or twisted due to fatigue during the workout.

We have learned that Dynamic Stretching is moving a limb through its full range of motion at various speeds, and that it is more efficient at improving both static and dynamic flexibility than static stretching.

And we have learned that PNF stretching is very fast and efficient at improving both range of motion and motor performance in a short period of time, which is very motivating.

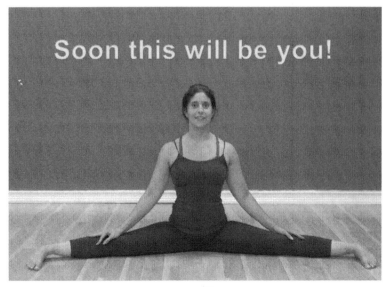

6

So, what is this method, what does it consist of, how often do we do it, when do we do it, etc?

So far, we've learned about three types of stretching,

Static, **Dynamic**, and **PNF**.

In this method of achieving the splits and high kicks quickly, safely and properly, we use a carefully designed combination of **Advanced Dynamic Stretching** with Stops and **PNF Stretching** which has been proven to give the fastest and most efficient results.

As I mentioned before, everything from:

> ➢ how many reps you do,
> ➢ how many seconds you hold a stretch,
> ➢ how often you do it,
> ➢ when you do it,

all these things have been researched and tested so that every detail that I'm giving you here has been maximized for best results and efficiency.

Static stretching, the common kind which we've learned should be done at the end of workouts, is not really a part of this program, it's just sort of optional or supplemental.

Dynamic and **PNF** methods will form the bulk of the program. It is likely that, since you are doing this course, you are involved in regular athletic activity of some kind. Whether it be gymnastics, cheer-leading, dance, weightlifting or martial arts, you can and should do some static stretching at the end of your activity period, for the reasons discussed in the previous section. But that is not really part of this program.

The Stretching Scientifically Program:

➢ Dynamic Stretching (leg swinging with stops) will be done five days per week in the mornings

➢ Dynamic Stretching session will take only approximately 10 minutes in the morning

➢ (Optional) -Evening Dynamic Stretching session - 10 min

➢ PNF-Contract/Relax/Extend Stretching will be done three days per week in the evenings

➢ PNF-Contract-Relax/Extend Stretching will take 10-15 minutes maximum

➢ Two days off per week

That's it! You don't have to spend two hours stretching every day to reach your maximum potential. It can be done in just minutes a day.

So, the most obvious and efficient schedule for most people looks like this:

Sunday	Monday	Tuesday	Wednesday	Thursday	Friday	Saturday
Evening (Rest)	PNF Stretching		PNF Stretching		PNF Stretching	Evening (Rest)
Morning (Rest)	Dynamic Stretching	Dynamic Stretching	Dynamic Stretching	Dynamic Stretching	Dynamic Stretching	Morning (Rest)

I have reproduced this on the following page in a larger format so that you can photocopy it if you like.

Stretching Scientifically Schedule

Sunday	Monday	Tuesday	Wednesday	Thursday	Friday	Saturday
Evening Rest	PNF Stretching		PNF Stretching		PNF Stretching	Evening Rest
Morning Rest	Dynamic Stretching	Dynamic Stretching	Dynamic Stretching	Dynamic Stretching	Dynamic Stretching	Morning Rest

7

Introduction to Dynamic Stretching Routine

In Chapter 3, I introduced you to the basic principles of dynamic stretching.

Dynamic stretching is the first way we use to reprogram the nervous system.

As you may recall, we are going to do our dynamic stretching in the morning, shortly after awakening, to reprogram our body for movement.

You see, your body is always trying to adapt to whatever you do, and if you sleep 7 or 8 hours like most people do, your body has been lying relatively still for a long period of time, one third of the 24 hours in a day. During that time, your muscles, although relaxed in some fashion, tend to shorten and tighten up.

That is why it we do dynamic stretching in the morning, to reset the nervous system and inform the body that we would like a full range of motion to be available for our daily activities.

So, you want to do your dynamic stretching routine in the morning after awakening as soon as possible, but you must allow your muscles to warm up first. Remember, we don't stretch cold muscles, and by "cold" we mean inactive muscles that haven't moved in a while.

In this sequence, I will instruct you to warm up the hamstrings with some butt kicks (explained in the next section) before you begin your first leg swinging exercise, but you can also go for a walk or morning run before doing your Dynamic Stretches if you so choose.

The Dynamic Stretches are done in 3 sets of 12 to 16 repetitions, similar to a weightlifting routine.

In the first set of each exercise, we move relatively slowly and in a controlled fashion through a near full range of movement for 12 to 16 repetitions, depending on your energy level and what feels right to you that day.

Then, in the second set, we increase the velocity of our swinging a bit and make sure we go to both ends of the range of motion, stopping the motion of the leg with our hands or a kicking pad.

In the third set, we move our hands an inch or two higher than their previous position and perform the exercise with maximum velocity and enthusiasm, making sure that we solidly stop the swinging of the limb with our hands or a padded object. This is what encourages the muscles to lengthen and relax.

You will notice right away that the ease of performing the stretching exercise and your range of motion increase with each set. As the days and weeks go by, the difference becomes more pronounced. You might eventually begin your first set swinging your leg waist high, your second set shoulder high, and your third set over your head.

With continued practice, you can usually reach the point where you will only need to do one set, with say, five repetitions slow and easy, five medium, then five full blast.

If you get lazy and stop doing your morning stretches, your flexibility will diminish. Remember, your body is constantly trying to adapt to what you do, and if you do nothing, well, that's what you are telling your body that you want to do.

But don't worry if you messed up for a while, it comes back real fast. Just do your best to be as regular as possible with your stretching routine if you want fast and amazing results.

8

How To: Front Leg Swing

The front leg swing is our first Dynamic Stretching exercise.

It can be performed in various fashions, but before performing any variation, make sure you have sufficiently warmed up the hamstring muscles on the back of the leg. You can warm up the legs by walking or jogging for 5 to 10 minutes, or you can just do a few minutes of butt-kicking.

Butt- Kicking

To perform the Butt-Kicking hamstring warm-up, simply place your hands on your hips and alternately contract your hamstrings, shifting your weight to one leg and bringing your opposite heel up to your buttocks.

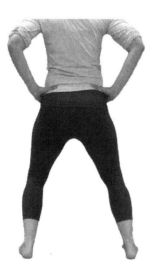 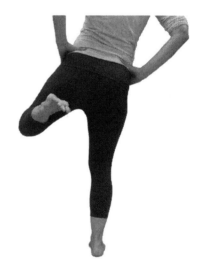

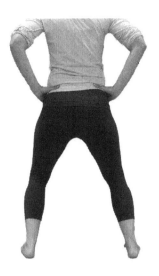 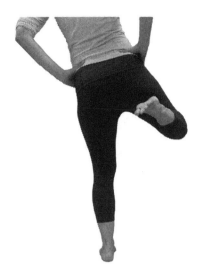

Return the foot to the floor and contract the opposite side in a rhythmic manner, for 20 or 30 repetitions.

The Front Leg Swing-Version 1

Once the hamstrings are warmed up, you can begin the first set of front leg swings.

The first version to be presented will be the Front Leg Swing utilizing the Wall.

One aligns themselves an arm's length away from a wall and places their palm on the wall or alternatively holds on to a pole, bar or chair as shown in the illustrations.

The leg closest to the wall is the one that will be swung while the remaining leg supports the weight of the body.

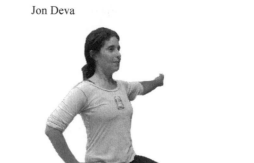
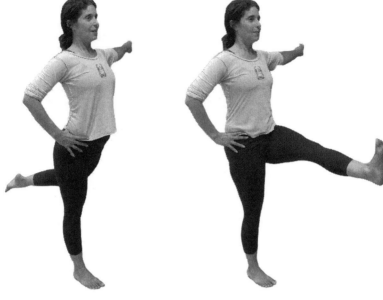

In the first set of swings, begin by swinging the leg from the hip to the front and back in a slow and relaxed manner, keeping the leg straight, to about 80%-90% of its full range of motion, allowing the hip joint to open and become well lubricated. After 12 to 16 repetitions, repeat on the other side.

It can be very useful and comfortable if the supporting leg can be placed on a brick or a block, which elevates the entire body creating plenty of space for the leg to swing, but this is not necessary.

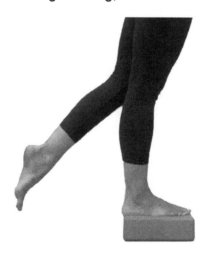

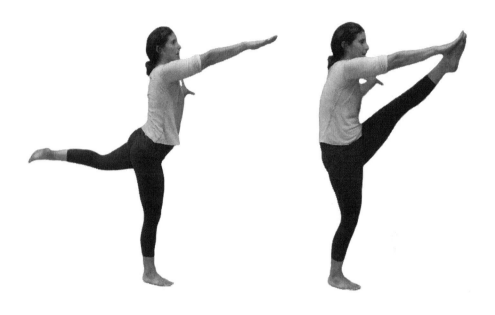

Now begin the second set. In the second set, we increase the speed a bit and make sure to go to the full end of the current range of motion, stopping the motion of swinging leg firmly with our free hand.

If you are unable to put any strength into your hand to stop the swinging leg, it will serve no purpose and you will get better results by having someone else hold a kicking pad or padded object to stop the swinging leg.

After 12 to 16 repetitions, whatever feels right to you, repeat on the opposite side.

Now for the third and final set, place your free hand or padded object an inch or two higher than it was during the second set and begin swinging your leg up quite rapidly to be stopped by the waiting hand or pad. This is where you give it your all.

Perform 12 to 16 repetitions and repeat on the other side.

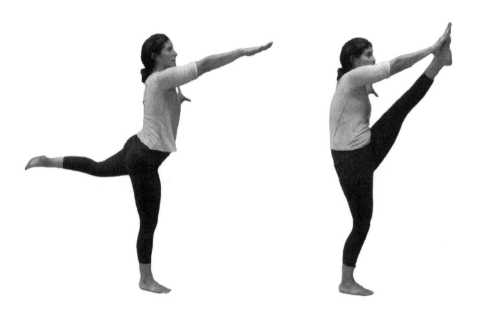

Congratulations, you have finished three sets of front leg swings utilizing the wall! This is the preferred technique for front leg swings to be use in the morning session.

About the Breathing

During the first set of legs swings, as it is done in quite a relaxed manner, you just breath normally. During the second and third sets, however, you should exhale as the leg rises up and inhale as it goes back down.

Front Leg Swing Variations

The two following variations on the front leg swing may be preferred by martial artists or those who don't have sufficient strength in one hand to stop the swinging leg completely.

Both of the following variations utilize both hands to stop the swinging leg, which tends to give the leg muscles more confidence that the leg will be stopped and thus it relaxes more, increasing your range of motion.

The Front Leg Swing-Version 2

In version two of the front leg swing, you start in a standard martial arts style front stance position, with one leg bent in front and the other extended and straight behind you as shown. Both hands are extended to the front to stop the swinging leg.

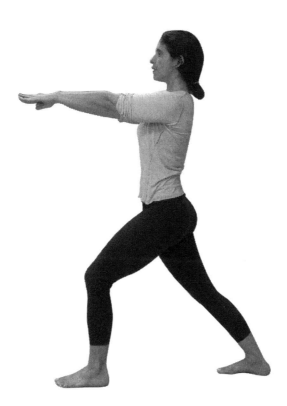

You then rise up on the front leg, swinging the rear leg to the front and stopping the leg with both hands.

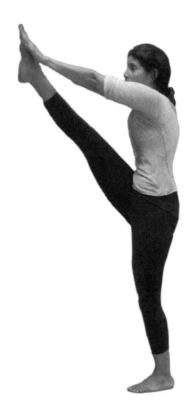

The swinging leg may be stopped at the instep or shin, depending upon your current level of flexibility and comfort.

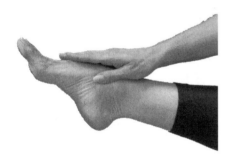 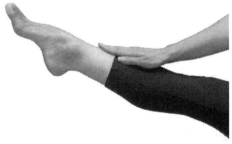

Allow the leg to swing back down and return it to the starting position in the rear.

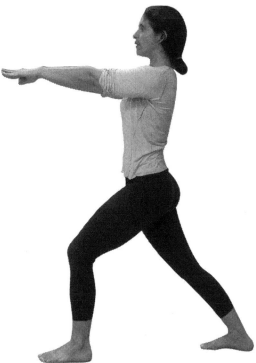

Perform your 12 to 16 repetitions on one side, then the other.

Remember to begin gently, increasing the speed and range of motion with each set.

The Front Leg Swing-Version 3

Version three of the front leg swing is similar to version two, the only difference being that instead of placing the swinging leg back down to the rear, we place it in front and then kick with the opposite leg.

This causes us to move forward, alternately stepping and swing-kicking the leg. This version can be performed when there is plenty of space to move forward and is ideal, but not necessary.

Versions One and Two can be performed in a limited amount of space and will give great results.

29

9

How To: Side Leg Swing

The side leg swing is our second Dynamic Stretching exercise.

Unlike the front leg swing, which seems quite easy and natural due to its similarity to our everyday walking motion, the side leg swing can feel quite awkward at first and one should be quite careful and controlled when first learning this motion.

Unless you are a dancer, gymnast or martial artist, it is unlikely that your body is accustomed to moving in this fashion, so do start slowly and give yourself time to adjust.

Do not be overzealous with this one or you will be likely to hurt yourself. Injury must be avoided at all costs, so give your body all the time it needs to adapt to this movement. If you do things correctly, it won't take long at all.

To perform the side leg swing dynamic stretching exercise, it is best to grab a bar, heavy chair or support of some kind with the hand opposite the side of the swinging leg as shown in the photo.

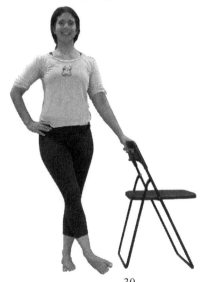

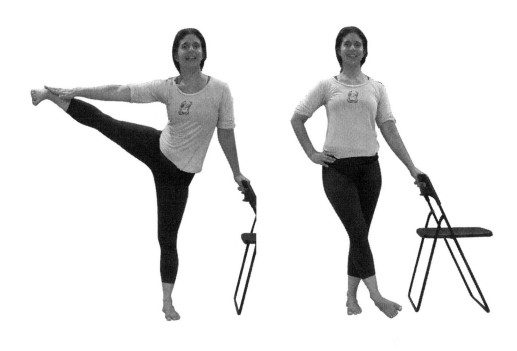

As in the front leg swing, begin by swinging the leg from the hip to the side and up in a slow and relaxed manner, keeping the leg straight, to about 80%-90% of its full range of motion.

In the first set, it's just lifting and opening the leg to the side. The muscles on the side of the hip are usually quite weak at first, so don't shoot for 16 repetitions if you find yourself feeling tired or strained at 12. Just take it easy and warm up the joint in this direction.

In the second and third sets of the side swing, you will add more speed and make sure to stop the leg at or near the end of its range of motion with the free hand.

Many people find themselves bending forward at the waist as the leg comes up higher and higher to the side. This is ok. In some athletic disciplines, you may want to work toward a more upright position over time, but bending forward in the beginning is acceptable.

Just like the Front leg swings, you want to work your way up to three sets of 12-16 repetitions, however, if you find your hips weak at first, just do one set for the first week, then two the second week, if you feel ready, and so on.

10

How To: Back Leg Swing

The back leg swing is our third and final Dynamic Stretching exercise.

It is different from the first two Dynamic Stretches in the following respects:

There is no stopping of the swinging leg with the hand.
The body is bent parallel to the ground and not held upright.
The base leg is actually the leg being most stretched.

The back leg swing begins by placing both hands on a stable surface at an appropriate height such as a chair, as shown in the photo.

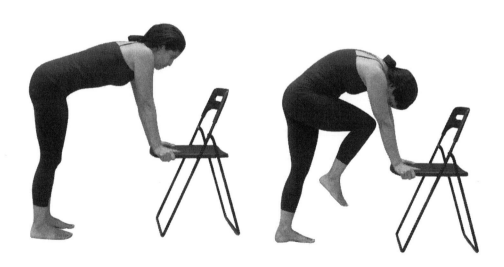

The torso is held parallel to the floor and one knee is brought forward to the chest, then the leg is brought down, out and up in an arc to the rear with the toes pointed down.

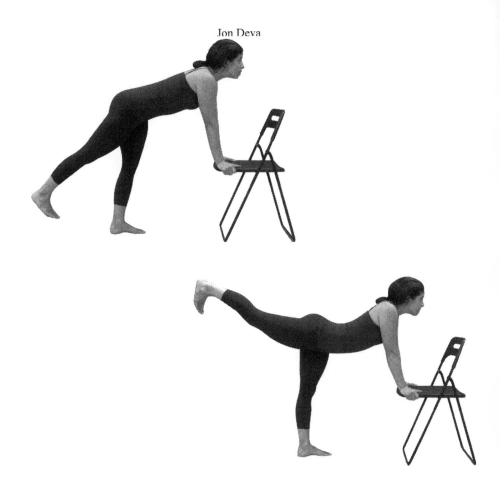

The head should be looking forward as the leg arcs upward to the rear. A powerful stretch will be felt in the muscles of the base leg if the exercise is performed properly.

Beginners, however, usually perform this exercise incorrectly, pointing the toes to the side, opening the hip.

Check yourself carefully in the beginning, to make sure you are performing the exercise correctly, with the hips square and the toes pointed down, and you will get fast results.

You can perform One to Three sets of this exercise.

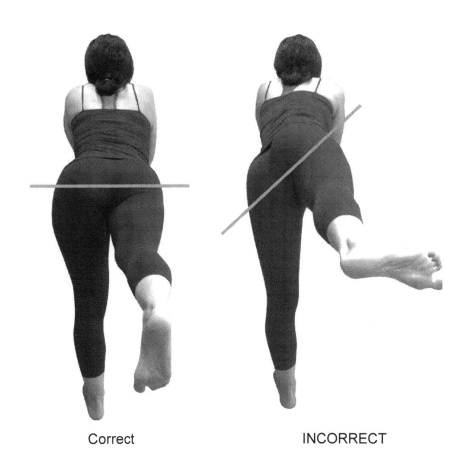

Correct   INCORRECT

Summary- Dynamic Stretching Routine

So now you've learned the details of how to do the Front, Side, and Back leg swings.

Ideally, you'll be performing these Dynamic Stretches five days a week, preferably in the morning, after a quick warm up, to reprogram your body for movement.

If you are unable to do these in the morning, because you have to rush off to school or work or whatever, It's ok. You can do them in the afternoon or evening also. But it's best to do them in the morning.

You will notice, if you do perform them in the afternoon or evening, that they will probably feel much easier and your range of motion might be greater than it is in the morning. That's normal, it's just because your muscles have had all day to warm up.

As stated in the program overview in Chapter 6, you can do an extra set of Dynamic stretches in the evening if you like, as part of your workout or training, but it is not required.

> You should begin this program by practicing these dynamic stretching exercises for at least a week or two before adding in the PNF stretching technique which is explained in the following sections.

You already know everything you need to know to get started, so mark your calendar and get to it!

You can study the following sections on PNF/Contract-Relax-Extend stretching during your first and second week of Dynamic Stretching, then add it into your routine 3 times a week when you feel ready.

11

Defining the Splits

Before we begin

Before we begin explaining the specific details of PNF stretching for the front and side splits, it is important to clearly define what the front and side splits actually are.

There are actually three types of splits commonly practiced, the front, side, and hurdler's split, sometimes called the open front split.

Side Split

The side split, or straddle as it is sometimes called, is relatively simple to define, as each leg rotates out from the hip directly to the left and right sides of the body, with the legs eventually forming one line perpendicular to the torso. The feet can remain flat on the ground, or pointing out to the sides, or the toes may be pointed up, the torso maybe upright or on the ground, all of these are still the side split.

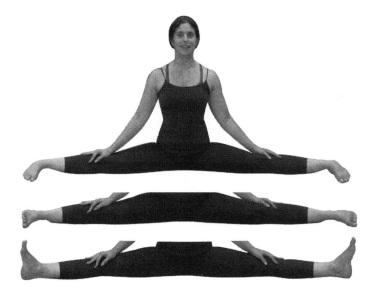

Front Split

In the front split, or true front split as it is sometimes called, one leg rotates from the hip directly to the front of the body with toes pointing forward or upward, while the other goes directly behind, with the hips square and the front side of the rear leg in contact with the ground as shown. The instep or toes of the rear foot will be pointed down.

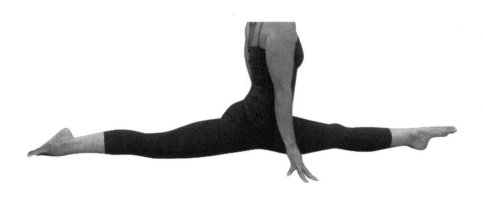

Hurdler's Split

The hurdler's split is what you get when most people try to do the front splits. The front leg goes out just the same, but due to a lack of frontal hip flexibility, the rear leg has the side of the leg in contact with the ground instead of the front, and the hips are not square. Basically, if the toes of the rear leg are pointed to the side, it's a hurdler's split and not a front split.

As the hurdler's split is just an open front split, or a front split with the hips unsquared and the side of the rear leg on the ground, no specific training will be done for this split. As you work on your side split and front split, a hurdler's split will come about easily and naturally, with no specific effort required.

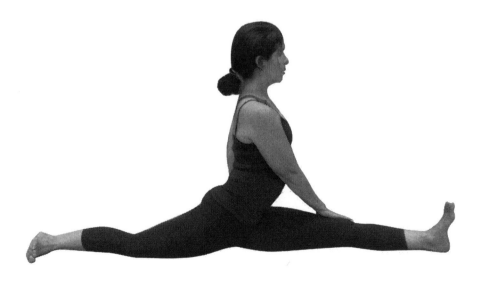

Jon Deva

12

PNF for Side Splits

And now the fun begins!

If you want to follow my system exactly, before beginning PNF Stretching for the side splits, you should have been performing at least two weeks of dynamic stretching. If you have done so, you have most certainly already noticed gains in your range of motion and the speed at which your muscles go from "stiff" to "warmed-up".

It is now time to add PNF Stretching into the program.

How to do PNF for Side Splits:

PNF Stretching for the side splits is relatively simple. As you recall from the explanatory section on PNF Stretching, the method requires you simply move a limb to the end of its current range of motion and then add specific cycles of contraction and relaxation of the muscles being stretched.

So, in the case of the side splits, we begin in standing position and lower ourselves to approximately 90% or 95% of our maximum stretch, and then attempt to squeeze the legs together for about 8-10 seconds.

Pressing down and pinching the ground between your legs as if you could squeeze the earth up between your legs. Then relax the muscles completely for 20-30 seconds, supporting your weight on chairs or the ground if necessary.

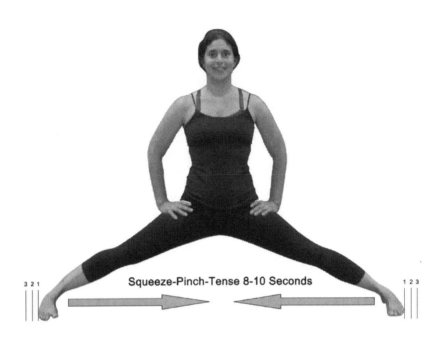

3 2 1 Squeeze-Pinch-Tense 8-10 Seconds 1 2 3

At this point, you usually find that your range of motion has increased a little, so you extend the stretch a little further and begin the cycle again.

This is repeated a total of 3 times.

1: Stretch - Contract 8-10 seconds – Relax 20-30 seconds – Extend Range of Motion a little bit.

2: Stretch - Contract 8-10 seconds – Relax 20-30 seconds – Extend Range of Motion a little bit.

3: Stretch - Contract 8-10 seconds – Relax 20-30 seconds – Extend Range of Motion a little bit.

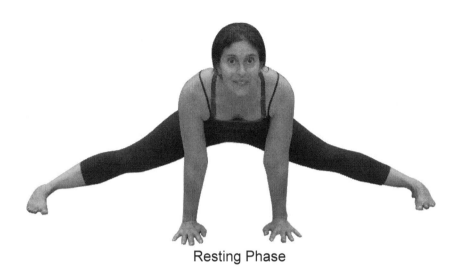

Resting Phase

After completing three these three cycles of contraction, relaxation and stretching, drop to the ground and finish with your normal straddle stretching routine.

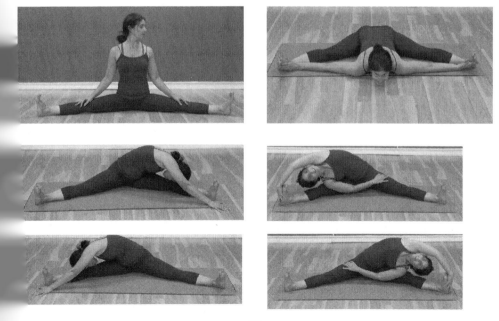

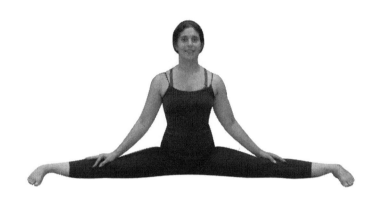

With continued practice, you will reach the full straddle.

Important:

If you wish to incorporate the PNF stretching into your current gymnastics or martial arts or dance workouts, you MUST add them in at the END of your routine, that is, after all other workout activities have been performed. Never follow PNF Stretching with any attempt at athletic activity. Static stretching alone is permitted after PNF.

I repeat: If you are going to incorporate the PNF stretching into a current workout routine, it is exceedingly important that they be the last thing that you do, in the cool-down period, as they can severely diminish proprioception (motor-skill-coordination) for a short period of time after the performance of the technique.

(Translation: Your legs will be wobbly and you will most likely injure yourself if you try anything athletic after PNF Stretching).

Strength:

In the beginning, you will most likely lack strength in the standing side split and need to support yourself on chairs, or lean over and support your torso with your extended arms on the floor, especially during the 20-30 second "rest" period between cycles. This weakness will quickly diminish and in a short period of time you will find that you can do all three cycles of contraction without needing to support yourself with chairs or the floor.

. Notes:

> During the 8-10 second contraction, the muscle should be contracted only to 50% to 75% of full tension. Do not contract maximally.

> There is (usually) no benefit in repeating the cycle more than three times. Occasionally, you may experiment with five cycles instead of three.

> Sometimes, your muscles will be tight and refuse to extend. Do not force increased range of motion.

> **PNF Stretching** is only to be done 3 times per week.

> **PNF Stretching** will produce some amount of muscle soreness on the following day. You should know that you stretched the night before, but you should not be in pain and unable to walk. If so, you over did it!

13

PNF for Front Splits

Now that you have learned PNF stretching for the side splits, you should have a fairly good idea of what is involved in doing PNF stretching for the front splits. It is only slightly more complicated.

Due to the fact that the limiting factor on the front splits is always the limited flexibility of the front hip of the rear leg, that is where we place most of the emphasis when training for the full front split.

Begin by assuming a long lunge position as shown in the photograph.

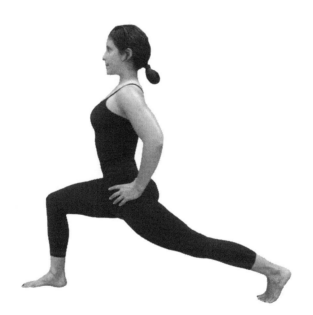

At first we are going to warm-up and pre exhaust the front hip muscles by holding this lunge position with the rear leg locked as straight as possible for one minute. Some lifting and lowering of the pelvis a few inches is permissible during this period, but the rear leg is kept tight and straight.

If one minute is impossible for you, you can begin with 30 seconds, but work your way to a minute as soon as possible.

After the one minute hold, lower your rear knee gently to the floor.
It is preferable to use a pad or folded towel under then knee so that you can be comfortable and concentrate on stretching the hip.

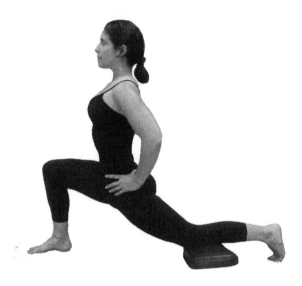

Once you have assumed this position, you can relax into the posture for the next 30 seconds to one minute, allowing your hips to sink as low as possible. You can also gently lean backward, stretching the front of the hip in a normal passive static manner.

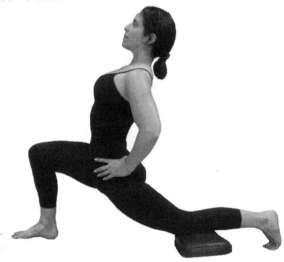

Returning your torso to a vertical position, extend your front leg a bit until your shin is at approximately a 45 degree angle as shown.

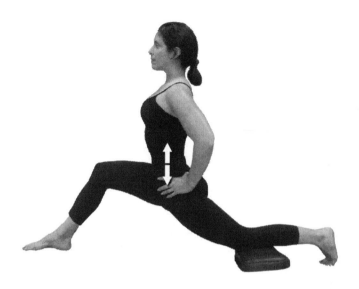

We are now ready to begin the PNF portion of the stretching segment. Simply contract the muscles of the rear leg as if you were trying to bring the knee forward, but without letting it move. At the same time contract the muscles of the front leg back toward the knee as if you were trying to pinch the earth between your front leg and your knee.

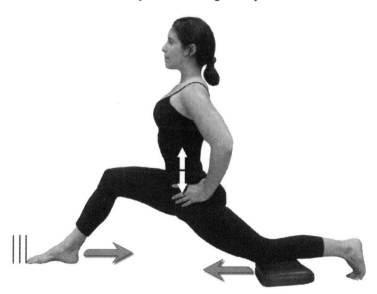

Hold the contraction for 8-10 seconds, then relax the muscles completely for 20-30 seconds, supporting your weight on chairs or the ground if necessary. Extend your front foot a little bit forward, and repeat the cycle two more times.

Obviously, as you become stronger and more flexible over time, you can allow yourself to go further and further into the front split, while maintaining the same feeling of contracting your muscles and pinching the earth up between your thighs.

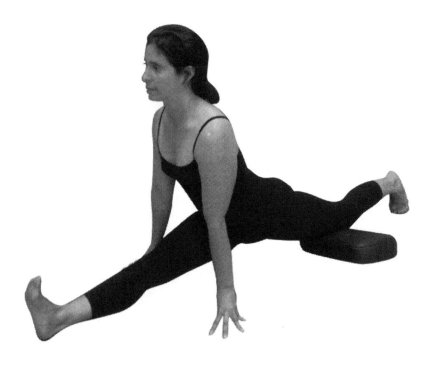

And that's all there is too it!

You now know how to do PNF stretching for both the side and front splits and if you follow the program carefully, respecting your limitations, not trying too hard and just following the program schedule, you will find your flexibility increasing like never before.

Remember:

➢ During the 8-10 second contraction, the muscle should be contracted only to 50% to 75% of full tension. Do not contract maximally.

➢ There is (usually) no benefit in repeating the cycle more than three times. Occasionally, you may experiment with five cycles instead of three.

➢ Sometimes, your muscles will be tight and refuse to extend. Do not force increased range of motion.

➢ **PNF Stretching** is only to be done 3 times per week.

➢ **PNF Stretching** will produce some amount of muscle soreness on the following day. You should know that you stretched the night before, but you should not be in pain and unable to walk. If so, you over did it!

Printed in Great Britain
by Amazon